I0415556

Blood Pressure and Pulse Logbook For Monitoring Heart Health

Dubreck World Publishing

Copyright

'Blood Pressure and Pulse Logbook For Monitoring Heart Health'

First published in July 2021 by Dubreck World Publishing
Printed and bound by Lulu Press
Distributed by Lulu Press

Copyright © 2021 Dubreck World Publishing, Hampshire, UK

ISBN-13: 978-1-105-71179-4

First Edition

DUBRECK WORLD PUBLISHING

Blood Pressure Monitoring

Regularly record your blood pressure and pulse in this logbook and take it with you to your next doctor or nurse appointment. This will help them see your overall progress and consider if any adjustment to your treatment may be necessary.

Record your blood pressure as often as you are advised to by a qualified medical practitioner.

Understanding Your Blood Pressure

Taking your blood pressure is a way of measuring the strength with which the blood pushes the sides of your arteries as the heart pumps it around your body.

Checking your blood pressure will show you if it is high (hypertension), normal, or low (hypotension). Low blood pressure can cause dizziness and fainting, and long term high blood pressure can cause serious complications, as shown in the diagram on the next page.

If you suffer with high hypertension, your medical practitioner may advise you to regularly check your blood pressure and record your results.

30 minutes before checking your blood pressure, don't exercise, smoke, drink caffeine or eat a big meal as these may elevate your results. You should also empty your bladder at least five minutes before taking a reading.

Try and measure your blood pressure at the same times each day and take two or three readings each time, one minute apart and then log each reading in your log book.

When you take your blood pressure, you will have two readings. The systolic number is the higher number. This measures the pressure of the blood in your arteries when your heart beats. The diastolic number is the lower number. This measures the pressure of the blood in your arteries when your heart rests in between beats.

Main complications of persistent
High blood pressure

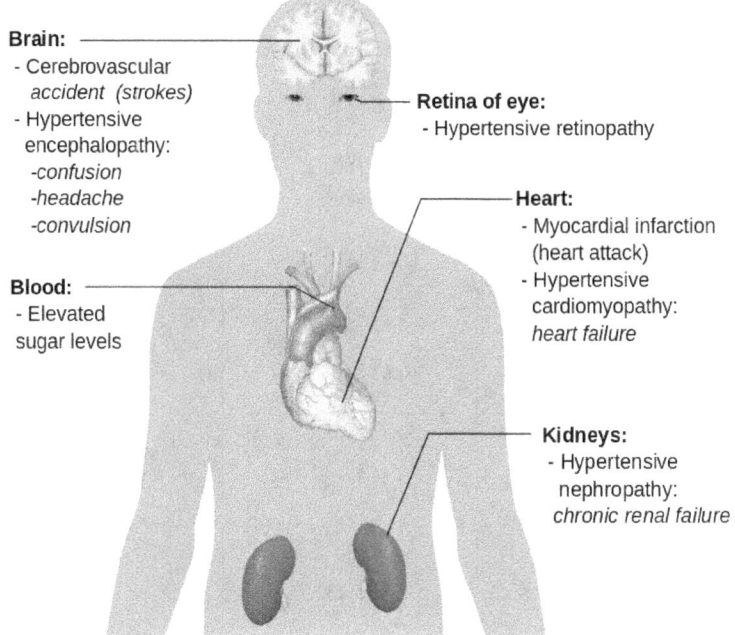

Brain:
- Cerebrovascular
  accident (strokes)
- Hypertensive
  encephalopathy:
  -confusion
  -headache
  -convulsion

Blood:
- Elevated
  sugar levels

Retina of eye:
- Hypertensive retinopathy

Heart:
- Myocardial infarction
  (heart attack)
- Hypertensive
  cardiomyopathy:
  heart failure

Kidneys:
- Hypertensive
  nephropathy:
  chronic renal failure

What Should Your Blood Pressure Be?

Category	Systolic BP mmHg	Diastolic BP mmHg
Optimal	<120	<80
Normal	120-129	80-84
High Normal	130-139	85-89
Grade 1 Hypertension	140-159	90-99
Grade 2 Hypertension	160-179	100-109
Grade 3 Hypertension	>180	>110

These are based on blood pressure levels for adults.

Personal Details

Personal

Name_____

Address_____

_____

_____

Tel_____

Email_____

D.O.B._____

Medical

Doctor's Name_____

Doctor's Surgery_____

Doctor's Tel_____

Emergency Contact

First Contact:

Name_____

Phone_____

Second Contact:

Name_____

Phone_____

Blood Pressure and Pulse Log

Example

Date	Time	Blood Pressure	Pulse
26/7/21	8.30am	123/82	77
		/	
		/	
Notes			
Feeling well			

Date	Time	Blood Pressure	Pulse
		/	
		/	
		/	

Notes

Date	Time	Blood Pressure	Pulse
		/	
		/	
		/	

Notes

Date	Time	Blood Pressure	Pulse
		/	
		/	
		/	

Notes

Date	Time	Blood Pressure	Pulse
		/	
		/	
		/	
Notes			

Date	Time	Blood Pressure	Pulse
		/	
		/	
		/	
Notes			

Date	Time	Blood Pressure	Pulse
		/	
		/	
		/	
Notes			

Date	Time	Blood Pressure	Pulse
		/	
		/	
		/	
Notes			

Date	Time	Blood Pressure	Pulse
		/	
		/	
		/	
Notes			

Date	Time	Blood Pressure	Pulse
		/	
		/	
		/	
Notes			

Date	Time	Blood Pressure	Pulse
		/	
		/	
		/	
Notes			

Date	Time	Blood Pressure	Pulse
		/	
		/	
		/	
Notes			

Date	Time	Blood Pressure	Pulse
		/	
		/	
		/	
Notes			

Date	Time	Blood Pressure	Pulse
		/	
		/	
		/	
Notes			

Date	Time	Blood Pressure	Pulse
		/	
		/	
		/	
Notes			

Date	Time	Blood Pressure	Pulse
		/	
		/	
		/	
Notes			

Date	Time	Blood Pressure	Pulse
		/	
		/	
		/	
Notes			

Date	Time	Blood Pressure	Pulse
		/	
		/	
		/	
Notes			

Date	Time	Blood Pressure	Pulse
		/	
		/	
		/	
Notes			

Date	Time	Blood Pressure	Pulse
		/	
		/	
		/	
Notes			

Date	Time	Blood Pressure	Pulse
		/	
		/	
		/	
Notes			

Date	Time	Blood Pressure	Pulse
		/	
		/	
		/	
Notes			

Date	Time	Blood Pressure	Pulse
		/	
		/	
		/	

Notes

Date	Time	Blood Pressure	Pulse
		/	
		/	
		/	

Notes

Date	Time	Blood Pressure	Pulse
		/	
		/	
		/	

Notes

Date	Time	Blood Pressure	Pulse
		/	
		/	
		/	

Notes

Date	Time	Blood Pressure	Pulse
		/	
		/	
		/	

Notes

Date	Time	Blood Pressure	Pulse
		/	
		/	
		/	

Notes

Date	Time	Blood Pressure	Pulse
		/	
		/	
		/	
Notes			

Date	Time	Blood Pressure	Pulse
		/	
		/	
		/	
Notes			

Date	Time	Blood Pressure	Pulse
		/	
		/	
		/	
Notes			

Date	Time	Blood Pressure	Pulse
		/	
		/	
		/	
Notes			

Date	Time	Blood Pressure	Pulse
		/	
		/	
		/	
Notes			

Date	Time	Blood Pressure	Pulse
		/	
		/	
		/	
Notes			

Date	Time	Blood Pressure	Pulse
		/	
		/	
		/	
Notes			

Date	Time	Blood Pressure	Pulse
		/	
		/	
		/	
Notes			

Date	Time	Blood Pressure	Pulse
		/	
		/	
		/	
Notes			

Date	Time	Blood Pressure	Pulse
		/	
		/	
		/	
Notes			

Date	Time	Blood Pressure	Pulse
		/	
		/	
		/	
Notes			

Date	Time	Blood Pressure	Pulse
		/	
		/	
		/	
Notes			

Date	Time	Blood Pressure	Pulse
		/	
		/	
		/	

Notes

Date	Time	Blood Pressure	Pulse
		/	
		/	
		/	

Notes

Date	Time	Blood Pressure	Pulse
		/	
		/	
		/	

Notes

Date	Time	Blood Pressure	Pulse
		/	
		/	
		/	

Notes

Date	Time	Blood Pressure	Pulse
		/	
		/	
		/	

Notes

Date	Time	Blood Pressure	Pulse
		/	
		/	
		/	

Notes

Date	Time	Blood Pressure	Pulse
		/	
		/	
		/	
Notes			

Date	Time	Blood Pressure	Pulse
		/	
		/	
		/	
Notes			

Date	Time	Blood Pressure	Pulse
		/	
		/	
		/	
Notes			

Date	Time	Blood Pressure	Pulse
		/	
		/	
		/	

Notes

Date	Time	Blood Pressure	Pulse
		/	
		/	
		/	

Notes

Date	Time	Blood Pressure	Pulse
		/	
		/	
		/	

Notes

Date	Time	Blood Pressure	Pulse
		/	
		/	
		/	

Notes

Date	Time	Blood Pressure	Pulse
		/	
		/	
		/	

Notes

Date	Time	Blood Pressure	Pulse
		/	
		/	
		/	

Notes

Date	Time	Blood Pressure	Pulse
		/	
		/	
		/	

Notes

Date	Time	Blood Pressure	Pulse
		/	
		/	
		/	

Notes

Date	Time	Blood Pressure	Pulse
		/	
		/	
		/	

Notes

Date	Time	Blood Pressure	Pulse
		/	
		/	
		/	
Notes

Date	Time	Blood Pressure	Pulse
		/	
		/	
		/	
Notes

Date	Time	Blood Pressure	Pulse
		/	
		/	
		/	
Notes

Date	Time	Blood Pressure	Pulse
		/	
		/	
		/	

Notes

Date	Time	Blood Pressure	Pulse
		/	
		/	
		/	

Notes

Date	Time	Blood Pressure	Pulse
		/	
		/	
		/	

Notes

Date	Time	Blood Pressure	Pulse
		/	
		/	
		/	

Notes

Date	Time	Blood Pressure	Pulse
		/	
		/	
		/	

Notes

Date	Time	Blood Pressure	Pulse
		/	
		/	
		/	

Notes

Date	Time	Blood Pressure	Pulse
		/	
		/	
		/	

Notes

Date	Time	Blood Pressure	Pulse
		/	
		/	
		/	

Notes

Date	Time	Blood Pressure	Pulse
		/	
		/	
		/	

Notes

Date	Time	Blood Pressure	Pulse
		/	
		/	
		/	

Notes

Date	Time	Blood Pressure	Pulse
		/	
		/	
		/	

Notes

Date	Time	Blood Pressure	Pulse
		/	
		/	
		/	

Notes

Date	Time	Blood Pressure	Pulse
		/	
		/	
		/	

Notes

Date	Time	Blood Pressure	Pulse
		/	
		/	
		/	

Notes

Date	Time	Blood Pressure	Pulse
		/	
		/	
		/	

Notes

Date	Time	Blood Pressure	Pulse
		/	
		/	
		/	
Notes			

Date	Time	Blood Pressure	Pulse
		/	
		/	
		/	
Notes			

Date	Time	Blood Pressure	Pulse
		/	
		/	
		/	
Notes			

Date	Time	Blood Pressure	Pulse
		/	
		/	
		/	

Notes

Date	Time	Blood Pressure	Pulse
		/	
		/	
		/	

Notes

Date	Time	Blood Pressure	Pulse
		/	
		/	
		/	

Notes

Date	Time	Blood Pressure	Pulse
		/	
		/	
		/	
Notes			

Date	Time	Blood Pressure	Pulse
		/	
		/	
		/	
Notes			

Date	Time	Blood Pressure	Pulse
		/	
		/	
		/	
Notes			

Date	Time	Blood Pressure	Pulse
		/	
		/	
		/	

Notes

Date	Time	Blood Pressure	Pulse
		/	
		/	
		/	

Notes

Date	Time	Blood Pressure	Pulse
		/	
		/	
		/	

Notes

Date	Time	Blood Pressure	Pulse
		/	
		/	
		/	

Notes

Date	Time	Blood Pressure	Pulse
		/	
		/	
		/	

Notes

Date	Time	Blood Pressure	Pulse
		/	
		/	
		/	

Notes

Date	Time	Blood Pressure	Pulse
		/	
		/	
		/	

Notes

Date	Time	Blood Pressure	Pulse
		/	
		/	
		/	

Notes

Date	Time	Blood Pressure	Pulse
		/	
		/	
		/	

Notes

Date	Time	Blood Pressure	Pulse
		/	
		/	
		/	
Notes			

Date	Time	Blood Pressure	Pulse
		/	
		/	
		/	
Notes			

Date	Time	Blood Pressure	Pulse
		/	
		/	
		/	
Notes			

Date	Time	Blood Pressure	Pulse
		/	
		/	
		/	

Notes

Date	Time	Blood Pressure	Pulse
		/	
		/	
		/	

Notes

Date	Time	Blood Pressure	Pulse
		/	
		/	
		/	

Notes

Date	Time	Blood Pressure	Pulse
		/	
		/	
		/	

Notes

Date	Time	Blood Pressure	Pulse
		/	
		/	
		/	

Notes

Date	Time	Blood Pressure	Pulse
		/	
		/	
		/	

Notes

Date	Time	Blood Pressure	Pulse
		/	
		/	
		/	
Notes			

Date	Time	Blood Pressure	Pulse
		/	
		/	
		/	
Notes			

Date	Time	Blood Pressure	Pulse
		/	
		/	
		/	
Notes			

Date	Time	Blood Pressure	Pulse
		/	
		/	
		/	
Notes			

Date	Time	Blood Pressure	Pulse
		/	
		/	
		/	
Notes			

Date	Time	Blood Pressure	Pulse
		/	
		/	
		/	
Notes			

Date	Time	Blood Pressure	Pulse
		/	
		/	
		/	

Notes

Date	Time	Blood Pressure	Pulse
		/	
		/	
		/	

Notes

Date	Time	Blood Pressure	Pulse
		/	
		/	
		/	

Notes

Date	Time	Blood Pressure	Pulse
		/	
		/	
		/	
Notes			

Date	Time	Blood Pressure	Pulse
		/	
		/	
		/	
Notes			

Date	Time	Blood Pressure	Pulse
		/	
		/	
		/	
Notes			

Date	Time	Blood Pressure	Pulse
		/	
		/	
		/	

Notes

Date	Time	Blood Pressure	Pulse
		/	
		/	
		/	

Notes

Date	Time	Blood Pressure	Pulse
		/	
		/	
		/	

Notes

Date	Time	Blood Pressure	Pulse
		/	
		/	
		/	

Notes

Date	Time	Blood Pressure	Pulse
		/	
		/	
		/	

Notes

Date	Time	Blood Pressure	Pulse
		/	
		/	
		/	

Notes

Date	Time	Blood Pressure	Pulse
		/	
		/	
		/	

Notes

Date	Time	Blood Pressure	Pulse
		/	
		/	
		/	

Notes

Date	Time	Blood Pressure	Pulse
		/	
		/	
		/	

Notes

Date	Time	Blood Pressure	Pulse
		/	
		/	
		/	

Notes

Date	Time	Blood Pressure	Pulse
		/	
		/	
		/	

Notes

Date	Time	Blood Pressure	Pulse
		/	
		/	
		/	

Notes

Date	Time	Blood Pressure	Pulse
		/	
		/	
		/	

Notes

Date	Time	Blood Pressure	Pulse
		/	
		/	
		/	

Notes

Date	Time	Blood Pressure	Pulse
		/	
		/	
		/	

Notes

Date	Time	Blood Pressure	Pulse
		/	
		/	
		/	

Notes

Date	Time	Blood Pressure	Pulse
		/	
		/	
		/	

Notes

Date	Time	Blood Pressure	Pulse
		/	
		/	
		/	

Notes

Date	Time	Blood Pressure	Pulse
		/	
		/	
		/	

Notes

Date	Time	Blood Pressure	Pulse
		/	
		/	
		/	

Notes

Date	Time	Blood Pressure	Pulse
		/	
		/	
		/	

Notes

Date	Time	Blood Pressure	Pulse
		/	
		/	
		/	
Notes			

Date	Time	Blood Pressure	Pulse
		/	
		/	
		/	
Notes			

Date	Time	Blood Pressure	Pulse
		/	
		/	
		/	
Notes			

Date	Time	Blood Pressure	Pulse
		/	
		/	
		/	

Notes

Date	Time	Blood Pressure	Pulse
		/	
		/	
		/	

Notes

Date	Time	Blood Pressure	Pulse
		/	
		/	
		/	

Notes

Date	Time	Blood Pressure	Pulse
		/	
		/	
		/	

Notes

Date	Time	Blood Pressure	Pulse
		/	
		/	
		/	

Notes

Date	Time	Blood Pressure	Pulse
		/	
		/	
		/	

Notes

Date	Time	Blood Pressure	Pulse
		/	
		/	
		/	

Notes

Date	Time	Blood Pressure	Pulse
		/	
		/	
		/	

Notes

Date	Time	Blood Pressure	Pulse
		/	
		/	
		/	

Notes

Date	Time	Blood Pressure	Pulse
		/	
		/	
		/	
Notes			

Date	Time	Blood Pressure	Pulse
		/	
		/	
		/	
Notes			

Date	Time	Blood Pressure	Pulse
		/	
		/	
		/	
Notes			

Date	Time	Blood Pressure	Pulse
		/	
		/	
		/	

Notes

Date	Time	Blood Pressure	Pulse
		/	
		/	
		/	

Notes

Date	Time	Blood Pressure	Pulse
		/	
		/	
		/	

Notes

Date	Time	Blood Pressure	Pulse
		/	
		/	
		/	
Notes			

Date	Time	Blood Pressure	Pulse
		/	
		/	
		/	
Notes			

Date	Time	Blood Pressure	Pulse
		/	
		/	
		/	
Notes			

Date	Time	Blood Pressure	Pulse
		/	
		/	
		/	

Notes

Date	Time	Blood Pressure	Pulse
		/	
		/	
		/	

Notes

Date	Time	Blood Pressure	Pulse
		/	
		/	
		/	

Notes

Date	Time	Blood Pressure	Pulse
		/	
		/	
		/	

Notes

Date	Time	Blood Pressure	Pulse
		/	
		/	
		/	

Notes

Date	Time	Blood Pressure	Pulse
		/	
		/	
		/	

Notes

Date	Time	Blood Pressure	Pulse
		/	
		/	
		/	
Notes			

Date	Time	Blood Pressure	Pulse
		/	
		/	
		/	
Notes			

Date	Time	Blood Pressure	Pulse
		/	
		/	
		/	
Notes			

Date	Time	Blood Pressure	Pulse
		/	
		/	
		/	

Notes

Date	Time	Blood Pressure	Pulse
		/	
		/	
		/	

Notes

Date	Time	Blood Pressure	Pulse
		/	
		/	
		/	

Notes

Date	Time	Blood Pressure	Pulse
		/	
		/	
		/	

Notes

Date	Time	Blood Pressure	Pulse
		/	
		/	
		/	

Notes

Date	Time	Blood Pressure	Pulse
		/	
		/	
		/	

Notes

Date	Time	Blood Pressure	Pulse
		/	
		/	
		/	
Notes			

Date	Time	Blood Pressure	Pulse
		/	
		/	
		/	
Notes			

Date	Time	Blood Pressure	Pulse
		/	
		/	
		/	
Notes			

Date	Time	Blood Pressure	Pulse
		/	
		/	
		/	

Notes

Date	Time	Blood Pressure	Pulse
		/	
		/	
		/	

Notes

Date	Time	Blood Pressure	Pulse
		/	
		/	
		/	

Notes

Date	Time	Blood Pressure	Pulse
		/	
		/	
		/	

Notes

Date	Time	Blood Pressure	Pulse
		/	
		/	
		/	

Notes

Date	Time	Blood Pressure	Pulse
		/	
		/	
		/	

Notes

Date	Time	Blood Pressure	Pulse
		/	
		/	
		/	

Notes

Date	Time	Blood Pressure	Pulse
		/	
		/	
		/	

Notes

Date	Time	Blood Pressure	Pulse
		/	
		/	
		/	

Notes

Date	Time	Blood Pressure	Pulse
		/	
		/	
		/	

Notes

Date	Time	Blood Pressure	Pulse
		/	
		/	
		/	

Notes

Date	Time	Blood Pressure	Pulse
		/	
		/	
		/	

Notes

Date	Time	Blood Pressure	Pulse
		/	
		/	
		/	
Notes			

Date	Time	Blood Pressure	Pulse
		/	
		/	
		/	
Notes			

Date	Time	Blood Pressure	Pulse
		/	
		/	
		/	
Notes			

Date	Time	Blood Pressure	Pulse
		/	
		/	
		/	
Notes			

Date	Time	Blood Pressure	Pulse
		/	
		/	
		/	
Notes			

Date	Time	Blood Pressure	Pulse
		/	
		/	
		/	
Notes			

Date	Time	Blood Pressure	Pulse
		/	
		/	
		/	

Notes

Date	Time	Blood Pressure	Pulse
		/	
		/	
		/	

Notes

Date	Time	Blood Pressure	Pulse
		/	
		/	
		/	

Notes

Date	Time	Blood Pressure	Pulse
		/	
		/	
		/	

Notes

Date	Time	Blood Pressure	Pulse
		/	
		/	
		/	

Notes

Date	Time	Blood Pressure	Pulse
		/	
		/	
		/	

Notes

Date	Time	Blood Pressure	Pulse
		/	
		/	
		/	

Notes

Date	Time	Blood Pressure	Pulse
		/	
		/	
		/	

Notes

Date	Time	Blood Pressure	Pulse
		/	
		/	
		/	

Notes

Date	Time	Blood Pressure	Pulse
		/	
		/	
		/	

Notes

Date	Time	Blood Pressure	Pulse
		/	
		/	
		/	

Notes

Date	Time	Blood Pressure	Pulse
		/	
		/	
		/	

Notes

Date	Time	Blood Pressure	Pulse
		/	
		/	
		/	
Notes			

Date	Time	Blood Pressure	Pulse
		/	
		/	
		/	
Notes			

Date	Time	Blood Pressure	Pulse
		/	
		/	
		/	
Notes			

Date	Time	Blood Pressure	Pulse
		/	
		/	
		/	

Notes

Date	Time	Blood Pressure	Pulse
		/	
		/	
		/	

Notes

Date	Time	Blood Pressure	Pulse
		/	
		/	
		/	

Notes

Date	Time	Blood Pressure	Pulse
		/	
		/	
		/	

Notes

Date	Time	Blood Pressure	Pulse
		/	
		/	
		/	

Notes

Date	Time	Blood Pressure	Pulse
		/	
		/	
		/	

Notes

Date	Time	Blood Pressure	Pulse
		/	
		/	
		/	
Notes			

Date	Time	Blood Pressure	Pulse
		/	
		/	
		/	
Notes			

Date	Time	Blood Pressure	Pulse
		/	
		/	
		/	
Notes			

Date	Time	Blood Pressure	Pulse
		/	
		/	
		/	

Notes

Date	Time	Blood Pressure	Pulse
		/	
		/	
		/	

Notes

Date	Time	Blood Pressure	Pulse
		/	
		/	
		/	

Notes

Date	Time	Blood Pressure	Pulse
		/	
		/	
		/	
Notes			

Date	Time	Blood Pressure	Pulse
		/	
		/	
		/	
Notes			

Date	Time	Blood Pressure	Pulse
		/	
		/	
		/	
Notes			

Date	Time	Blood Pressure	Pulse
		/	
		/	
		/	

Notes

Date	Time	Blood Pressure	Pulse
		/	
		/	
		/	

Notes

Date	Time	Blood Pressure	Pulse
		/	
		/	
		/	

Notes

Date	Time	Blood Pressure	Pulse
		/	
		/	
		/	

Notes

Date	Time	Blood Pressure	Pulse
		/	
		/	
		/	

Notes

Date	Time	Blood Pressure	Pulse
		/	
		/	
		/	

Notes

Date	Time	Blood Pressure	Pulse
		/	
		/	
		/	

Notes

Date	Time	Blood Pressure	Pulse
		/	
		/	
		/	

Notes

Date	Time	Blood Pressure	Pulse
		/	
		/	
		/	

Notes

Date	Time	Blood Pressure	Pulse
		/	
		/	
		/	

Notes

Date	Time	Blood Pressure	Pulse
		/	
		/	
		/	

Notes

Date	Time	Blood Pressure	Pulse
		/	
		/	
		/	

Notes

Date	Time	Blood Pressure	Pulse
		/	
		/	
		/	

Notes

Date	Time	Blood Pressure	Pulse
		/	
		/	
		/	

Notes

Date	Time	Blood Pressure	Pulse
		/	
		/	
		/	

Notes

Date	Time	Blood Pressure	Pulse
		/	
		/	
		/	

Notes

Date	Time	Blood Pressure	Pulse
		/	
		/	
		/	

Notes

Date	Time	Blood Pressure	Pulse
		/	
		/	
		/	

Notes

Date	Time	Blood Pressure	Pulse
		/	
		/	
		/	

Notes

Date	Time	Blood Pressure	Pulse
		/	
		/	
		/	

Notes

Date	Time	Blood Pressure	Pulse
		/	
		/	
		/	

Notes

Date	Time	Blood Pressure	Pulse
		/	
		/	
		/	
Notes			

Date	Time	Blood Pressure	Pulse
		/	
		/	
		/	
Notes			

Date	Time	Blood Pressure	Pulse
		/	
		/	
		/	
Notes			

Date	Time	Blood Pressure	Pulse
		/	
		/	
		/	

Notes

Date	Time	Blood Pressure	Pulse
		/	
		/	
		/	

Notes

Date	Time	Blood Pressure	Pulse
		/	
		/	
		/	

Notes

Date	Time	Blood Pressure	Pulse
		/	
		/	
		/	
Notes			

Date	Time	Blood Pressure	Pulse
		/	
		/	
		/	
Notes			

Date	Time	Blood Pressure	Pulse
		/	
		/	
		/	
Notes			

Date	Time	Blood Pressure	Pulse
		/	
		/	
		/	

Notes

Date	Time	Blood Pressure	Pulse
		/	
		/	
		/	

Notes

Date	Time	Blood Pressure	Pulse
		/	
		/	
		/	

Notes

Date	Time	Blood Pressure	Pulse
		/	
		/	
		/	

Notes

Date	Time	Blood Pressure	Pulse
		/	
		/	
		/	

Notes

Date	Time	Blood Pressure	Pulse
		/	
		/	
		/	

Notes

Date	Time	Blood Pressure	Pulse
		/	
		/	
		/	

Notes

Date	Time	Blood Pressure	Pulse
		/	
		/	
		/	

Notes

Date	Time	Blood Pressure	Pulse
		/	
		/	
		/	

Notes

Date	Time	Blood Pressure	Pulse
		/	
		/	
		/	
Notes			

Date	Time	Blood Pressure	Pulse
		/	
		/	
		/	
Notes			

Date	Time	Blood Pressure	Pulse
		/	
		/	
		/	
Notes			

Date	Time	Blood Pressure	Pulse
		/	
		/	
		/	

Notes

Date	Time	Blood Pressure	Pulse
		/	
		/	
		/	

Notes

Date	Time	Blood Pressure	Pulse
		/	
		/	
		/	

Notes

Date	Time	Blood Pressure	Pulse
		/	
		/	
		/	

Notes

Date	Time	Blood Pressure	Pulse
		/	
		/	
		/	

Notes

Date	Time	Blood Pressure	Pulse
		/	
		/	
		/	

Notes

Date	Time	Blood Pressure	Pulse
		/	
		/	
		/	
Notes			

Date	Time	Blood Pressure	Pulse
		/	
		/	
		/	
Notes			

Date	Time	Blood Pressure	Pulse
		/	
		/	
		/	
Notes			

Date	Time	Blood Pressure	Pulse
		/	
		/	
		/	

Notes

Date	Time	Blood Pressure	Pulse
		/	
		/	
		/	

Notes

Date	Time	Blood Pressure	Pulse
		/	
		/	
		/	

Notes

Date	Time	Blood Pressure	Pulse
		/	
		/	
		/	

Notes

Date	Time	Blood Pressure	Pulse
		/	
		/	
		/	

Notes

Date	Time	Blood Pressure	Pulse
		/	
		/	
		/	

Notes

Date	Time	Blood Pressure	Pulse
		/	
		/	
		/	

Notes

Date	Time	Blood Pressure	Pulse
		/	
		/	
		/	

Notes

Date	Time	Blood Pressure	Pulse
		/	
		/	
		/	

Notes

Date	Time	Blood Pressure	Pulse
		/	
		/	
		/	

Notes

Date	Time	Blood Pressure	Pulse
		/	
		/	
		/	

Notes

Date	Time	Blood Pressure	Pulse
		/	
		/	
		/	

Notes

Date	Time	Blood Pressure	Pulse
		/	
		/	
		/	
Notes			

Date	Time	Blood Pressure	Pulse
		/	
		/	
		/	
Notes			

Date	Time	Blood Pressure	Pulse
		/	
		/	
		/	
Notes			

Date	Time	Blood Pressure	Pulse
		/	
		/	
		/	

Notes

Date	Time	Blood Pressure	Pulse
		/	
		/	
		/	

Notes

Date	Time	Blood Pressure	Pulse
		/	
		/	
		/	

Notes

Date	Time	Blood Pressure	Pulse
		/	
		/	
		/	
Notes			

Date	Time	Blood Pressure	Pulse
		/	
		/	
		/	
Notes			

Date	Time	Blood Pressure	Pulse
		/	
		/	
		/	
Notes			

Date	Time	Blood Pressure	Pulse
		/	
		/	
		/	

Notes

Date	Time	Blood Pressure	Pulse
		/	
		/	
		/	

Notes

Date	Time	Blood Pressure	Pulse
		/	
		/	
		/	

Notes

Date	Time	Blood Pressure	Pulse
		/	
		/	
		/	

Notes

Date	Time	Blood Pressure	Pulse
		/	
		/	
		/	

Notes

Date	Time	Blood Pressure	Pulse
		/	
		/	
		/	

Notes

Date	Time	Blood Pressure	Pulse
		/	
		/	
		/	

Notes

Date	Time	Blood Pressure	Pulse
		/	
		/	
		/	

Notes

Date	Time	Blood Pressure	Pulse
		/	
		/	
		/	

Notes

Date	Time	Blood Pressure	Pulse
		/	
		/	
		/	

Notes

Date	Time	Blood Pressure	Pulse
		/	
		/	
		/	

Notes

Date	Time	Blood Pressure	Pulse
		/	
		/	
		/	

Notes

Date	Time	Blood Pressure	Pulse
		/	
		/	
		/	

Notes

Date	Time	Blood Pressure	Pulse
		/	
		/	
		/	

Notes

Date	Time	Blood Pressure	Pulse
		/	
		/	
		/	

Notes

Date	Time	Blood Pressure	Pulse
		/	
		/	
		/	

Notes

Date	Time	Blood Pressure	Pulse
		/	
		/	
		/	

Notes

Date	Time	Blood Pressure	Pulse
		/	
		/	
		/	

Notes

Date	Time	Blood Pressure	Pulse
		/	
		/	
		/	

Notes

Date	Time	Blood Pressure	Pulse
		/	
		/	
		/	

Notes

Date	Time	Blood Pressure	Pulse
		/	
		/	
		/	

Notes

Date	Time	Blood Pressure	Pulse
		/	
		/	
		/	

Notes

Date	Time	Blood Pressure	Pulse
		/	
		/	
		/	

Notes

Date	Time	Blood Pressure	Pulse
		/	
		/	
		/	

Notes

Date	Time	Blood Pressure	Pulse
		/	
		/	
		/	

Notes

Date	Time	Blood Pressure	Pulse
		/	
		/	
		/	

Notes

Date	Time	Blood Pressure	Pulse
		/	
		/	
		/	

Notes

Date	Time	Blood Pressure	Pulse
		/	
		/	
		/	
Notes			

Date	Time	Blood Pressure	Pulse
		/	
		/	
		/	
Notes			

Date	Time	Blood Pressure	Pulse
		/	
		/	
		/	
Notes			

Date	Time	Blood Pressure	Pulse
		/	
		/	
		/	

Notes

Date	Time	Blood Pressure	Pulse
		/	
		/	
		/	

Notes

Date	Time	Blood Pressure	Pulse
		/	
		/	
		/	

Notes

Date	Time	Blood Pressure	Pulse
		/	
		/	
		/	

Notes

Date	Time	Blood Pressure	Pulse
		/	
		/	
		/	

Notes

Date	Time	Blood Pressure	Pulse
		/	
		/	
		/	

Notes

Date	Time	Blood Pressure	Pulse
		/	
		/	
		/	
Notes				

Date	Time	Blood Pressure	Pulse
		/	
		/	
		/	
Notes				

Date	Time	Blood Pressure	Pulse
		/	
		/	
		/	
Notes				

Date	Time	Blood Pressure	Pulse
		/	
		/	
		/	
Notes			

Date	Time	Blood Pressure	Pulse
		/	
		/	
		/	
Notes			

Date	Time	Blood Pressure	Pulse
		/	
		/	
		/	
Notes			

Date	Time	Blood Pressure	Pulse
		/	
		/	
		/	

Notes

Date	Time	Blood Pressure	Pulse
		/	
		/	
		/	

Notes

Date	Time	Blood Pressure	Pulse
		/	
		/	
		/	

Notes

Date	Time	Blood Pressure	Pulse
		/	
		/	
		/	
Notes			

Date	Time	Blood Pressure	Pulse
		/	
		/	
		/	
Notes			

Date	Time	Blood Pressure	Pulse
		/	
		/	
		/	
Notes			

Date	Time	Blood Pressure	Pulse
		/	
		/	
		/	

Notes

Date	Time	Blood Pressure	Pulse
		/	
		/	
		/	

Notes

Date	Time	Blood Pressure	Pulse
		/	
		/	
		/	

Notes

Date	Time	Blood Pressure	Pulse
		/	
		/	
		/	
Notes			

Date	Time	Blood Pressure	Pulse
		/	
		/	
		/	
Notes			

Date	Time	Blood Pressure	Pulse
		/	
		/	
		/	
Notes			

Date	Time	Blood Pressure	Pulse
		/	
		/	
		/	

Notes

Date	Time	Blood Pressure	Pulse
		/	
		/	
		/	

Notes

Date	Time	Blood Pressure	Pulse
		/	
		/	
		/	

Notes

Date	Time	Blood Pressure	Pulse
		/	
		/	
		/	

Notes

Date	Time	Blood Pressure	Pulse
		/	
		/	
		/	

Notes

Date	Time	Blood Pressure	Pulse
		/	
		/	
		/	

Notes

Date	Time	Blood Pressure	Pulse
		/	
		/	
		/	

Notes

Date	Time	Blood Pressure	Pulse
		/	
		/	
		/	

Notes

Date	Time	Blood Pressure	Pulse
		/	
		/	
		/	

Notes

Date	Time	Blood Pressure	Pulse
		/	
		/	
		/	
Notes			

Date	Time	Blood Pressure	Pulse
		/	
		/	
		/	
Notes			

Date	Time	Blood Pressure	Pulse
		/	
		/	
		/	
Notes			

Date	Time	Blood Pressure	Pulse
		/	
		/	
		/	

Notes

Date	Time	Blood Pressure	Pulse
		/	
		/	
		/	

Notes

Date	Time	Blood Pressure	Pulse
		/	
		/	
		/	

Notes

Date	Time	Blood Pressure	Pulse
		/	
		/	
		/	

Notes

Date	Time	Blood Pressure	Pulse
		/	
		/	
		/	

Notes

Date	Time	Blood Pressure	Pulse
		/	
		/	
		/	

Notes

Date	Time	Blood Pressure	Pulse
		/	
		/	
		/	
Notes			

Date	Time	Blood Pressure	Pulse
		/	
		/	
		/	
Notes			

Date	Time	Blood Pressure	Pulse
		/	
		/	
		/	
Notes			

Date	Time	Blood Pressure	Pulse
		/	
		/	
		/	

Notes

Date	Time	Blood Pressure	Pulse
		/	
		/	
		/	

Notes

Date	Time	Blood Pressure	Pulse
		/	
		/	
		/	

Notes

Date	Time	Blood Pressure	Pulse
		/	
		/	
		/	
Notes			

Date	Time	Blood Pressure	Pulse
		/	
		/	
		/	
Notes			

Date	Time	Blood Pressure	Pulse
		/	
		/	
		/	
Notes			

Date	Time	Blood Pressure	Pulse
		/	
		/	
		/	

Notes

Date	Time	Blood Pressure	Pulse
		/	
		/	
		/	

Notes

Date	Time	Blood Pressure	Pulse
		/	
		/	
		/	

Notes

Date	Time	Blood Pressure	Pulse
		/	
		/	
		/	

Notes

Date	Time	Blood Pressure	Pulse
		/	
		/	
		/	

Notes

Date	Time	Blood Pressure	Pulse
		/	
		/	
		/	

Notes

www.ingramcontent.com/pod-product-compliance
Lightning Source LLC
Chambersburg PA
CBHW072138280526
45788CB00002B/692

* 9 7 8 1 1 0 5 7 1 1 7 9 4 *